Your Hair Care Arsenal

25 Easy DIY Oil Infusion Recipes to Protect your Natural Hair

By B. CliShea

Your Hair Care Arsenal

25 Easy DIY Oil Infusion Recipes to Protect your Natural Hair.
By B. **CliShea**

First Edition

https://www.clishea.co

Cover & Interior layout design by Mariana Vidakovics De Victor

Images from: https://pixabay.com/

Thank you for purchasing my ebook. As a way of giving thanks, you will receive a free gift that we are giving away along with the purchase of this book. Just click on the link below to receive your free gift.

GET YOUR FREE GIFT[1]

THANK YOU!

CONTENTS

Introduction

We all have had bad hair days at one point in our life. Bad hair days happen but bad hair everyday can be a big problem.

According to Datamonitor, in 2015 alone, the global hair care segment spending reached to 50 billion dollars. The total organic hair care spending in the same year was estimated to be 10.6 billion dollars or roughly 21.2% of the total global spending.

The increased awareness of the harmful effects of chemical-based hair care products triggered a switch to organic based hair products by as much as 33%.

The estimated total spending on organic hair care products is expected to reach by 15.98 billion dollars by 2020. This means the organic hair care products spending is expected to increase 1 billion dollars on the average every year.

Why am I telling you all these numbers?

These numbers tell you how much attention is given to hair care and its maintenance and that the hair care experts are gearing towards the use of organic ingredients.

The use of organic ingredients is now leading the trend of research and development of haircare products. Sadly, organic-based products are quite expensive. The alternative is to create a hair care product recipe that everyone can do themselves without the added high cost.

One option is the use of herbal hair oil infusion, which can give both the benefits of using organic herbs and oil which can give your hair a healthy, shiny look.

Massaging oil onto your hair will help strengthen the strands and improve the quality of your hair. When the oil is infused with herbs, you also get the added benefits contained in each property of the herb like dandruff control, scalp treatment, controls premature graying, dry hair, and other hair and scalp problems.

This book intends to provide readers the following:

* Learn the importance of using organic ingredients instead of chemical-based ingredients
* Create their own hair care and hair treatment recipe using organic based ingredients
* Produce their own hair care product without the expensive cost of advertising that branded products employ
* Help readers get their dream of having a healthy, soft and lustrous hair

This book is designed to help readers have more deciding power over the products they use in caring and maintaining a healthy scalp and hair.

Soon, bad hair days will be a thing of the past!

Chapter 1
Hair Care 101

Statistics show that the global hair care market is estimated to reach 85.5 billion US dollars by the end of 2017, and is estimated to reach the 100 billion US dollar mark by the year 2023. That's a 15-billion US dollar increase or about 17% growth in six years.

Consumers are now more aware of the need and importance of hair styling and care and are looking for more hair care products.

The increased awareness of the bad effects of chemicals on hair led to the soaring popularity of herbal care products.

How important is it to give your hair proper care?

Importance of hair care

You have all heard the cliché "your hair is your crowning glory". Your hair can make you look attractive or unattractive depending on how you style it.

After a flawless skin, your hair plays an important role in your physical appearance. The style and cut of your hair can tell a lot about you as a person.

If you style your hair regularly, chances are your hair strands could become brittle and split. Some hair care products can cause dryness and scalp itchiness.

However, you can minimize damage to your hair by following these simple hair care regimen:

* Regularly wash your hair. When washing your hair, make sure that you massage your scalp to keep them clean and healthy. A clean and healthy scalp will make your hair healthy
* Choose the right hair care aid. A lot of hair care products contain harsh chemical ingredients that can damage your hair. It is important that you use products with natural-based ingredients.
* If you need to use a blow-dryer, put the setting on low heat to dry your hair to minimize heat damage
* Give your hair a break. With so many hair care products available in the market today, hair styling has been made easy. While it is understandable that you style your hair when you need to go out, you need to give your hair a break by going natural.
* Trim your hair. Your hair is like grass that grows over time and just like grass, it needs a good trimming every now and then to maintain its healthy ends.
* Feed your hair. Believe it or not, your hair needs sustenance. Protein, vitamins, and mineral-rich foods help your hair grow and develop.
* Lastly, give your hair a hot oil treatment. Pamper your hair by giving it a hot oil treatment to make your hair shiny and less prone to damage.

Unfortunately, styling your hair and the use of chemical-based styling aids can lead to hair damage and eventually hair loss.

Common hair problems

Whatever style of hair you may have, you cannot escape having a bad hair day at one point in your life.

Here are some of the most common hair problems that men and women alike suffer from every day if not at one point in their life.

* Dry, brittle hair is due to the lack of moisture in your hair can lead to other hair problems like split ends, falling hair or frizzy hair. This is normally caused by prolonged exposure to heat like the sun or electric styling tools.
* Limp hair, other than medical related reason is also caused by hair care products build up. If you are using shampoo or conditioner that is heavy on the hair, this will build up over time making your hair lifeless and without volume.
* Split ends are the most common hair problem. When your hair becomes dry and brittle, the hair cuticle is damaged, causing the ends to split. Excessive hair styling, blow drying, hair coloring and straightening are some of the major causes of split ends
* Dandruff and flaky scalp cause itchiness. Your scalp is where your hair is rooted. It is the bed of your hair and it needs proper washing and care just as much as your hair. Excessive use of chemical based hair care products can cause the skin on your scalp to dry leaving flakes to form. Lack of nutrients can also cause your scalp to get dry.
* Dull hair is due to lack of moisture in your hair. Lack of protein, vitamins, and minerals from eating the right food can cause to the lack of natural moisture and shine of your hair. Chemical build up from hair care products can also cause your hair to become dull and limp.
* Heat damaged hair is caused by prolonged exposure

to the sun and the excessive use of blow dryer. No matter how healthy your hair is, excessive exposure to heat can cause your hair to become dry and brittle. Eventually, this could lead to other hair problems.

* Gray hair appears as part of the signs of aging. But, younger folks may exhibit gray hair, too. Exposure to heat, smoke, dirt, and chemicals can cause your hair to get damaged and become gray. Lack of essential vitamins and minerals can also lead to gray hair. Medical conditions that require radiation treatment is also known to cause gray hair.

* Falling Hair or Hair Loss is another common problem. Falling hair is caused by using the wrong hair care product and unhealthy scalp. If you are under chemotherapy treatment, hair loss occurs due to the exposure to radiation. Other health conditions that can cause hair loss includes alopecia, severe infections, surgery and, using of antidepressants.

Hair and Scalp Treatments

Hair and scalp problems can be treated. If you want to maintain shiny, healthy hair, eat healthy. Food nourishes your entire body including your hair.

Avoid the use of chemical based hair care products. If you feel that your shampoo is causing your hair problem, switch to a different brand or type. The popularity of a brand is not a guarantee that it is a good product.

There are plenty of natural-based ingredients hair products in the market such as herbal hair oil infused products, although they can prove to be a bit expensive.

If you are keen on going natural, you can make your own herbal hair oil infusion and this book will teach you how.

Chapter 2
Using Herbal Hair Oil Infusion

Prolong use of chemical-based hair treatments can damage your hair severely. Natural ingredients are available but the cost varies depending on the brand.

This chapter will teach you everything you need to know about natural herbs and introduce you the basic essentials of herbal hair oil infusion, including some of the most common herbs for a healthier and shinier hair.

What is an herb?

Herbs are plants or parts of a plant that are valued for its medicinal, savory and aromatic qualities.

Different ways to prepare Herbs

There are many ways to prepare herbs. Preparation depends on how you want to use the resulting end product.

* **Tinctures.** The tincture is extracted using a water and alcohol solution to soak the herbs. Alcohol is used to preserve the active ingredient of the herb. The extracted solution is stored in a sterilized bottle. The tincture is mixed with water before drinking.
* **Decoctions.** A mixture of roots, barks, and berries boiled in water to extract the active ingredient. The concoction is strained and stored in sterilized water. This is taken either hot or cold like a juice.
* **Creams.** This is created by simmering herbs and oil

(or fat) for three hours. The liquid is then strained and
stored in a sterilized dark bottles.
   * **Ointments.** Herb and oil (or fat) are heated quickly in a
     double boiler then strained and solidified.
   * **Drink infusion.** Made by boiling herb to create tea.
   * **Oil infusion.** This is made by combining crushed herbs,
     preferably dry crushed herbs and oil. You can infuse
     the mixture under the sun or by using a double boiler.
   The oil infusion preparation is what this book will
focus on.

What is an Herbal Hair Oil Infusion?

Herbal hair oil infusion is simply mixing herbs and oil.
You can use either fresh herb or dried herb although it is
recommended to use dried herbs to avoid the bacteria
coming from the natural moisture of the fresh herb.

If you do not want the added work of straining the
infused oil, you can use essential oil although essential oil
is quite expensive.

Infusion is done by heating oil and herb using a solar
method or cooking method:

   * *Solar Method* - heating the mixture under the heat of
     the sun. This method is tedious because it takes longer
     for the oil and herb to infuse.
   * *Cooking Method* - heating the mixture in a double boiler
     using low fire until the infusion happens. This method
     is quicker and more efficient.

What are the components of an herbal hair oil infusion?
   The basic components of an herbal hair oil infusion are
   * dried herbs or ready made essential oil
   * carrier oil

Carrier oil and essential oil will be discussed further in the succeeding chapters.

To prepare your herbal oil infusion, keep in mind the following:

Choose your container. Make sure to use a clean and dry container for your infused oil. Sterilize your bottle and let it dry. The best containers are those using cork lids instead of metal lids to avoid rust.

Choose your herbs. Choose an herb based on how the resulting end product you want. Using dried herbs is better than using fresh herbs. Bacteria grow faster in fresh herbs because of the natural moisture in fresh plants.

Choose your carrier oil. Olive oil and Jojoba oil have the longest shelf life among the various carrier oil available. Almond Oil is a favorite among the carrier oil because of its sweet fragrant smell

The infusion can be done by the cold method, heating method or sun heat method.

Common herbs for hair and scalp treatment

There are many herbs but not all herbs contain properties that are helpful in caring for the hair. Herbs are usually associated with cooking to help add flavor to your food but some herbs associated with food are also good for your hair.

Here a few list of herbs that can aid you in your hair and scalp care:

Herb	Origin	Benefits to Hair
Lavender	Mediterranean, Middle East, India	• Hair growth • Soothes scalp infections
Rosemary	Mediterranean	• Hair growth • Delays early graying • Nourishes dry scalp • Controls dandruff
Lemongrass	India, Burma, Thailand, Sri Lanka	• Strengthens hair • Prevents hair loss • Treats scalp inflammation
Aloe Vera	North Africa	• Contains Aloenin that regenerate hair cells • Conditions hair • Helps hair growth and thickness
Basil	India	• Removes flakes/dandruff
Sage	Mediterranean	• Good for oily hair • Controls dandruff • Effective for scalp infection • Restores hair color
Chamomile	Romans, ancient Egypt	• Soothes the scalp • Conditions and softens hair • Strengthens scalp • Adds shine to fair and blond hair
Henna	Ancient Egypt, India	• Seals moisture in hair • Deep conditions hair • Natural dye • Coats hair shaft

Herb	Origin	Benefits to Hair
Yucca Root	North America, Mexico	• Natural cleansing and foaming agent • Soothes and nourishes the scalp • Prevents hair loss • Controls dandruff
Burdoch	Northern Asia, Europe	• Conditions dry hair and scalp • Conditions oily hair and scalp • Prevents hair loss • Smoothens tangles • Gives hair body and luster

These are just ten of the most easy to find herbs you can use. You can find these herbs in the supermarket or right in your garden.

Chapter 3
What are carrier oils?

Carrier oil is one of the most important ingredients in making an herbal hair oil infusion.

In this Chapter, I will discuss carrier oils, its properties, how it is extracted and its uses. I will also discuss some of the most common carrier oils that help keep your hair healthy and strong.

What are carrier oils?

Carrier oils are base oils or vegetable oils derived naturally from plant kernels like nuts, or from seeds, or other fatty parts of a plant.

Carrier oils go rancid over time and the aroma is not as overpowering as that of essential oil.

Carrier oils are also derived from animal fossils but it is not a suitable carrier for personal care and aromatherapy infusions. Although mineral oil is used in many beauty products and personal care like baby oil, it is not a suitable carrier oil.

What are Essential Fatty Acids

Your body naturally produces fatty acids to keep it healthy. Those that are not produced naturally by your body is obtained by eating healthy food. Fatty acids help keep the body healthy and maintain the natural moisture of your skin.

The two of the most essential fatty acids are the Alpha-Linolenic Acid and the Linoleic Acid.

What are the uses of carrier oil?

The basic role is to act as carrying agent or a diffuser for essential oil.

Essential oil is potent and can cause irritation in its purest form. Carrier oil is normally added to dilute the strong potency of the essential oil.

Carrier Oil Preparation

You can prepare carrier oil in three different ways:

* *Preparation by cold pressing.* This is the most common way of preparing carrier oil. The oil is extracted from the fatty portion of the botanical plant using a pressing machine and the natural heat generated by the friction from the machine.
* *Preparation by cold expeller pressed.* This method is similar to cold pressing with extra heat kept to a minimum. The cool condition is necessary to keep the natural nutrients in the oil.
* *Preparation by solvent extraction.* This process uses a solvent to extract the oil. Using this process destroys the natural nutrients and fatty acids of the oil, leaving just remnants of the solvent mix with your oil.

After extraction the property of the oil changes from a virgin, extra virgin, unrefined and refined:

* Unrefined carrier oil is filtered to remove small particles and dust without affecting the natural state of its fatty acids, vitamins, and nutrients. Unrefined oil is the best quality of oil.
* Refined or Fractionated Oil is made to extend the shelf life of the oil thus destroying the vitamins, nutrients and fatty acids in the oil.
* Virgin or extra virgin oil applies mainly to olive oil. Extra virgin oil is extracted by cold pressing the olives just once. If you want to extract more oil, you can cold press more than once to derive virgin oil.

Common carrier oils and their benefits

There are many plants and seeds that are rich in fatty acids and used as carrier oils but not all of them are good for your hair.

It is important to note that the absorption rate of the oil will help you determine which type of oil would be best suited for your type of skin.

Fast absorbing oils are good for oily skin, Average absorbing oils are better for normal skin, while the slow absorbing oil is suited for the dry and mature skin.

Below are a few of the most common carrier oils that you can use in preparing your herbal hair oil infusion.

Carrier Oil	Origin	Benefits to Hair	Absorption
Jojoba Oil	Southern Arizona, Southern California, Northwestern Mexico	•Dissolves excess sebum •Nourishes Dry scalp	•Average
Coconut Oil	Africa, Asia, Polynesia	•Good for Dry Hair •Controls split ends	•Slow
Olive Oil	Mediterranean, Greece	•Good for dry hair •Treats dandruff •Keeps hair shiny and manageable	•Slow
Sweet Almond Oil	China, Central Asia	•Good for dry hair •Nourishes and strengthens hair •Treats hair damage	•Slow
Apricot Oil	Armenia	•Good for oily hair and scalp •Stimulates hair growth •Prevents loss of hair and scalp moisture	•Fast
Avocado Oil	South Central Mexico	•Good for dry hair •Stimulates blood flow in scalp	•Slow

Carrier Oil	Origin	Benefits to Hair	Absorption
Argan Oil	Morocco	• Good for normal hair • Ideal hair conditioner • Leaves hair softer and shinier • Tames frizzy hair • Treats split ends	• Average
Grape-seed Oil	North America	• Hair growth • Good for oily hair and scalp • Leaves hair shiny and non-greasy	• Fast
Hazel Nut Oil	Rome	• Hair growth • Nourish hair and scalp • Stimulates hair follicles	• Fast
Sesame Oil	Africa, India	• Strengthen hair from roots to tip • Treats premature graying • Controls dandruff • Treats dry hair	• Average

Chapter 4
Using Essential Oils

Essential oils are believed to have originated from Ancient Egypt. The Egyptians have been known to use oils for beauty and embalming purposes.

This chapter, you will learn more about essential oils, its uses, and preparation. I will also discuss the pros and cons of using essential oil and the role of carrier oils in essential oils. I have also included a simple conversion guide in using essential oil including the most common essential oil for hair and scalp treatment.

What are essential oils?

Essential oils are extracted from roots, barks, leave, flowers, and other parts of a botanical plant.

What are the uses of essential oils?

Essential oils are used in various ways and purposes. Most essential oils contain healing, soothing and aesthetic properties either in its purest form or mixed with other oils.

Essential Oil for hair care use

* Cure dandruff
* Hair shampoo
* Hair conditioner
* Itchy Scalp
* Hair thickener

* Oily Hair
* Dry Hair

Other than hair care, essential oils may be used as:

All purpose use at home as:

* Deodorizer
* All purpose cleaner
* Mosquito repellant
* Food flavoring (like peppermint)

Medicinal use for:

* Indigestion
* Burns
* Coughs and sinusitis
* Headaches

Relaxation / Spa

* Detox
* Improved sleep
* Massage / Sauna

How are essential oils extracted?

According to the National Association of Holistic Aromatherpy (NAHA), pure essential oil is extracted using the following process:

* Distillation
* Cold Pressing or Expression
* Enfleurage
* Solvent Extraction
* CO_2 Extraction

Among these processes, distillation and Expression are the two most common ways of extracting pure essential oil.

Some people consider maceration or infusion as a process to extract essential oil. In a sense, infusion of an herb with a carrier oil will extract the essential oil of a plant but the use of carrier oil will dilute the essential oil so it can no longer be considered as pure essential oil.

Difference of distillation and expression method:

Distillation is the process of separating the organic compound of the plant using water through the process of vaporization and condensation.

There are three types of distillation, water distillation, steam distillation and the combination of water and steam distillation.

Expression or cold pressing is used particularly on citrus plants like lemon, lime, oranges, bergamot, and tangerine. In ancient times, cold pressing is a manual process of using a sponge to extract the essential oil.

In modern times, cold pressing is done using a process called ecuelle a piquer. The process involves the use of a container with spikes to prick and prod the plant until the essential oil is released.

What are the dangers of essential oils?

The use of essential oil is the best alternative for a lot of health care remedies because of its organic components. However, the use of essential oil is not without danger.

Improper use of essential oil can lead to some dangerous effects

* Some oils can cause discoloration and burning of your

skin. There are oils that have a reaction when exposed to sunlight and can cause allergy or skin disorder. Citrus oils and cumin oils are known to be photosensitive oils.
* Oils like peppermint and lemongrass oils when applied undiluted can cause skin irritation and itching.
* Sage and wintergreen oils even when diluted can cause adverse effects on babies and pregnant women.
* Essential oils are potential dangers to your pets.
* Essential oils are potent and can affect breathing if inhaled directly.
* Drinking essential oil, even if diluted with water can cause death to anyone allergic to it

Essential Oil Unit of Conversion

Below is the standard unit of conversion and dilution for essential oil. This chart will help you when you want to prepare your own herbal oil infusion recipe.

Milliliters (ml)	Ounces (oz)	Drops
1	0.033	20
3.75	1/8	75
5	1/6	100
7.5	1/4	150
10	1/3	200
15	1/2	300
30	1	600
60	2	1200
120	4	2400
180	6	3600
249	8	4800

The essential oil should only be 1% - 2% of your total finished mix.

Example, if you are using 1% dilution, just add 6 drops of essential oils to a 30 ml bottle of lotion.

30 ml = 600 drops

1% of 600 drops = 6 drops

Common Essential Oils For Hair And Scalp Treatment

There a lot of botanical plants you can use to extract essential oils from and most of them are use not just for hair and scalp treatment but for other purposes as well.

The most common herbs listed in Chapter 2 are some of the commonly used essential oils that can help give you healthy hair and scalp. You can use any of them or combine them to create your own recipe.

Here are the top four widely used essential oils that you should never go without:

Essential Oil	Origin	Benefits to hair
Lavender	Mediterranean, India	• Antiseptic and anti-inflammatory properties help treat scalp inflammation. • Nourish and soothe irritation against dry, flaky skin. • Controls dandruff • Reduces hair loss • Gives luster to hair
Rosemary	Mediterranean	• Healthier scalp and hair • Metabolic function which can help stimulate hair growth • Prevents hair loss • Strengthens hair • Treats alopecia areata – a well-known hair loss problem.
Ylang Ylang	Philippines	• Improves hair thickness • Reduces split ends • Makes hair fuller and stronger • Improves oil balance in the scalp
Chamomile	Rome, Ancient Egypt	• Fights scalp inflammation • Prevents hair loss • Treats itchy scalp

Chapter 5
DIY Herbal Oil Infusion Recipe for Regular Hair Treatment

This Chapter will give you DIY recipes of to create hair oil infusion used as a regular treatment for your hair. There are several ways to pamper your hair and this chapter will discuss the benefits of each and include easy DIY recipes

HOT OIL TREATMENT (3 RECIPES)

What is hot oil treatment?

Hot Oil treatment is commonly used to prevent damage to hair or to reduce damage to hair.

Hot oil is massaged gently all over the scalp, covering the roots and tips of your hair.

Benefits of Using Hot Oil Treatment

* Hot oil treatment conditions your hair, giving it a shinier and more vibrant color.

* It also helps treat hair damage caused by the sun and chemicals from chemical based products.
* Helps increase blood circulation
* Moisturize dry and brittle hair

How often should you have a hot oil treatment?

Hot oil treatment should be done once a week especially if you have dry and brittle hair.

Massage the hot oil and leave it on for 30 minutes or longer depending on the extent of damage on your hair.

Recipe 1

Coconut Hot Oil Treatment for Normal Hair

INGREDIENTS:
- 4 oz coconut oil
- 24 drops of Ylang Ylang oil

PREPARATION:
1. Boil water in a saucepan on high heat.
2. Reduce the heat to keep the water simmering.
3. Use 1% dilution, measure 24 drops of Ylang Ylang essential oil.
4. Mix the Ylang Ylang essential oil with 4 ounces of coconut oil in a heat proof container.

5. Place the heat proof container on the simmering water to infuse the oil.

6. Let the infused oil cool

7. Keep in an amber colored jar

APPLICATION:
* Pour about 6 tablespoons of the oil in a container.
* Heat the container in hot water. Do not boil, just heat until it feels warm when touched.
* Pour the warm oil to your scalp.
* Slowly massage the oil from your scalp to the tip of your hair until it is coated.
* Cover your head with a shower cap and leave it on for 30 minutes or overnight, for best results.
* Shampoo and rinse your hair thoroughly to remove excess oil.

STORAGE:
Store in an amber colored jar and keep in a dry cool storage

SHELF LIFE
Shelf life is 1 – 2 years if stored properly

Recipe 2

· ·

DIY Homemade Hot Oil Treatment

· ·

INGREDIENTS:
- 2 tablespoon olive oil
- 2 tablespoon avocado oil
- 2 teaspoon jojoba oil
- 2 small bunches of fresh rosemary
- 6 to 8 drops of peppermint essential oil

PREPARATION:
1. Boil water in a medium saucepan.
2. Reduce to low heat to simmer water.
3. Mix olive oil, avocado oil, jojoba oil in a heat proof bowl.
4. Add the fresh rosemary but make sure the herb is dry and has no moisture.
5. Place the heat proof bowl over the simmering water.
6. Infuse for 30 minutes.
7. Check constantly to avoid drying up.
8. After infusing the oil and the herb, let it cool a little, but make sure it is still warm when you add the peppermint.
9. Add the peppermint essential oil drops.
10. Transfer the infused oil in an air tight container.

APPLICATION:
   * Cover your shoulder with a towel to keep your shirt
     clean.
   * Pour half of the oil mixture in a container.
   * Dip your fingers into the oil then apply it on your scalp.
   * Gently massage the oil from scalp to tip.
   * Coat your hair with the oil mixture.
   * Cover your head with a shower cap. For a better result,
     you can add a hot towel to cover your head before
     putting on the shower cap.
   * Shampoo hair and then rinse thoroughly.
   * Repeat the process once every 2 to 4 weeks.

STORAGE:
   * Store the oil in a heatproof and airtight container
   * Let the oil mixture cool first before closing the lid
   * Store in a dark cool place

SHELF LIFE:
   Shelf life is 2 to 4 weeks. Use of fresh herb can shorten
the shelf life of infused oils

Recipe 3

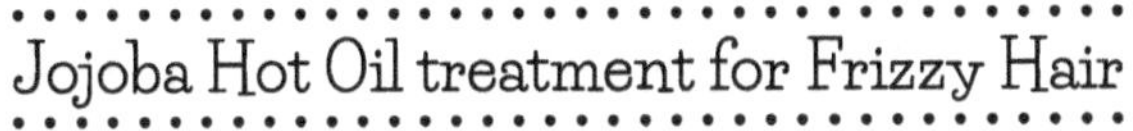

INGREDIENTS:
   * 2 tablespoon jojoba oil
   * 2 tablespoon argan oil
   * 6 drops of burdoch oil

PREPARATION:

1. Boil hot water in a saucepan in high heat.
2. Reduce the heat to keep the water simmering.
3. Mix jojoba oil, argan oil and burdoch oil in a heatproof container.
4. Place the heat proof container on the simmering water to infuse the oil.
5. Let the infused oil cool.
6. Keep in an amber colored jar.

APPLICATION:

* Pour about half of the oil in a container.
* Heat the container in hot water. Do not boil, just heat until it feels warm to the touch.
* Pour the warm oil to your scalp.
* Slowly massage the oil from your scalp to the tip of your hair until it is coated.
* Cover your head with a shower cap and leave it on for 30 minutes or overnight
* Shampoo and rinse your hair thoroughly to remove excess oil.

STORAGE:

* Store in an amber colored jar and keep in a dry cool storage
* Shelf life
* Shelf life is 1 – 2 years if stored properly

DEEP CONDITIONER TREATMENT (3 RECIPES)

Shampooing cleans your hair but daily use of shampoo can strip your hair of its natural shine and softness. To keep your hair smooth, soft and shiny you need to use a conditioner.

What is deep conditioner treatment?

Deep conditioning treatment is done to restore the strength and health of your hair. It allows your hair to withstand the stress of everyday styling and constant hair coloring.

Benefits of using deep conditioner treatment

Some of the benefits of using deep conditioner treatment are:

* Protects your hair from possible damages, like split ends, drying, breakage and brittleness.
* Helps retain the natural moisture of your hair to keep it healthy and strong
* Helps soften your hair, leaving it shiny and silky

How often should you have a deep conditioner treatment?

Deep conditioning should be done one to two times a week, three times if you have damaged or dry hair.

Recipe 1

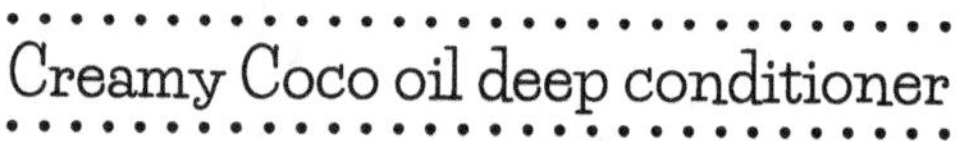

INGREDIENTS:
- 2 tablespoon coconut oil
- 1 tablespoon jojoba oil
- 3 – 5 drops of Lavender essential oil (or your own choice of essential oil)

PREPARATION:
1. Solidify your coconut oil by leaving it in the fridge for a few minutes.
2. Take 2 tablespoons of solid coconut oil and stir it in a bowl until it melts into a creamy state.
3. Add the jojoba oil and continue to stir until both oils are well combined.
4. Add the drops of lavender essential oil.
5. Stir well until the mixture is well combined.

APPLICATION:
* Dip your finger in the bowl and scoop up the creamy oil texture

* Gently massage your fingers all over your scalp, spreading the oil mixture from the roots to the tip of the hair.
* Give particular attention to the dry areas in you scalp.
* Once your hair is coated with the mixture, cover your head with a shower cap or a cling wrap plastic.
* You can put a warm towel under the cap or use a hair dryer to add some heat.
* Leave the oil mixture on your hair for 15-30 minutes.
* Rinse off the oil by washing and conditioning your hair.
* Repeat the process once a week.

STORAGE

You can make just enough of this mixture for one-time use, but if you have excess mixture, you can keep it in the fridge to keep the coconut oil solid.

SHELF LIFE

Since coconut oil has long shelf life, this should last until your next application.

Recipe 2

Coconut Oil deep hair conditioner

INGREDIENTS:

* 3 tablespoons coconut oil
* 1 tablespoon olive oil
* 8 drops Ylang Ylang essential oil
* Stand or hand mixer

PREPARATION:

1. Combine coconut oil, olive oil and essential oils in a mixing bowl.

2. Using a mixer, mix in medium/high speed all ingredients for 5 minutes or until the mixture becomes thick and creamy.

APPLICATION:

* Apply the whipped mixture onto your clean dry hair.
* Use a comb to spread the mixture evenly on your hair.
* Let it sit for 15-20 minutes.
* Rinse and shampoo afterward.
* Repeat once a week or as often as you wish.

STORAGE:

* Just prepare enough for one use. The creamy mixture will turn into foam, making it difficult to put in a bottle.
* Do not let the mixture sit in the sun.

SHELF LIFE:

Not advisable to be stored.

Will last as long as the oil with the shortest expiration.

Recipe 3

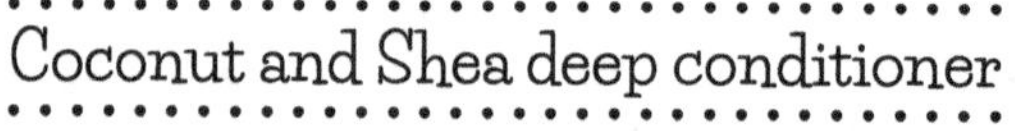

INGREDIENTS:

* 2 tablespoons coconut oil
* 1 tablespoon shea butter .
* 1 teaspoon argan oil
* 2 to 3 drops of Rosemary essential oil

PREPARATION:
1. Measure coconut oil and shea butter in solid form.
2. Melt the solid form in a microwave or a double broiler.
3. Wait until the mixture cools and becomes creamy.
4. Add the argan oil and the drops of rosemary essential oil.
5. Whip for 3 minutes or until you get a creamy consistency.

APPLICATION:
* Apply the mixture on your hair.
* Comb through to spread the mixture.
* Let it sit for 30 minutes.
* Shampoo hair, then rinse thoroughly.

STORAGE:
Just prepare enough mixture for one application so the mixture will not melt.

SHELF LIFE:
Not advisable for storage.

"PRE-POO" HAIR OIL TREATMENT (3 RECIPES)

Shampoo leaves residue that makes your hair heavy and dull. Harsh properties in shampoo can take away the luster and shine of your hair.

This is why some people added the pre-poo hair treatment as part of their hair care routine.

What is "pre-poo" hair oil treatment?

Pre-poo or Pre-shampoo treatment is a hair care practice done to prevent stripping your hair of its natural moisture and oils because of constant shampooing.

The treatment used is usually their favorite oil, hair masks, conditioner and DIY home treatments.

Benefits of using "pre-poo" hair oil treatment

Using pre-poo hair oil treatment can give your hair the following benefits:

* Restore your hair's moisture
* Restore your hair's shine
* Protects your hair from shampoo's harsh properties
* Soften your hair
* You get all the added benefits contained in the pre-poo treatment you are using.

How often should you have a "pre-poo" hair oil treatment?

You can do pre-poo hair oil treatment one to two times a week.

Recipe 1

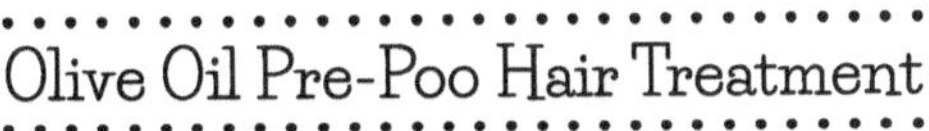

INGREDIENTS:
- ¼ cup Virgin olive oil
- 2 tablespoon castor oil
- 4 drops tea tree essential oil

PREPARATION:
1. Dilute tea tree essential oil with virgin olive oil and castor oil in a spritzer.
2. Mix and shake the oil mixture well.

APPLICATION:
* Spray the oil mixture from the roots of your hair to the tip.
* Cover your hair with a shower cap for 15 minutes or longer.
* Remove the shower cap and massage your scalp.
* Rinse and shampoo your hair.
* Repeat process once a week or as necessary.

STORAGE:
Keep in a spritzer for easy application on your hair

One application only.

Recipe 2

. . . .
Avocado Mask
. . . .

INGREDIENTS:
* One small ripe avocado
* 1 tablespoon coconut oil
* 1 tablespoon castor oil
* 1 tablespoon olive oil

PREPARATION:
1. Mash the ripe avocado until it becomes thick and creamy in consistency.
2. Add the coconut, castor, and olive oils.
3. Mix until all the oil is blended.
4. (Optional) You can heat in low fire to make it thicker.

APPLICATION:
* Apply the creamy mixture on your hair starting from roots to the tip.
* Leave it on overnight.
* Cover your head with a shower cap.
* Shampoo and then rinse thoroughly, to remove the avocado residue

STORAGE:
Make sure you use a small avocado that is only good for one application since the avocado tends to spoil.

SHELF LIFE:
  One application only

Recipe 3

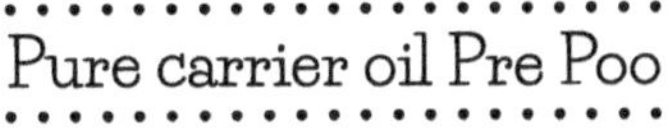

INGREDIENTS:
  - 2 tablespoon olive oil
  - 2 tablespoon castor oil
  - 2 tablespoon almond oil

PREPARATION:
  1. Mix the oils together in a spritzer.
  2. Shake well.

APPLICATION:
  * Spray on the oil mixture from the roots of your hair to the tip.
  * Cover your hair with a shower cap for 15 minutes or longer.
  * Remove the shower cap and massage your scalp.
  * Shampoo hair and rinse thoroughly.
  * Apply once a week.

STORAGE:
  Keep in a spritzer bottle

SHELF LIFE:
  Will last the same as the oil with the shortest shelf life

LEAVE-IN HAIR OIL TREATMENT (2 RECIPES)

When you talk about leave in hair treatment, it usually refers to leave on conditioners

What is leave in hair oil treatment?

Leave in hair oil treatment are conditioners sprayed on the hair usually to tame frizzy hairs.

Benefits of using leave-in hair oil treatment:

A good leave in conditioner can help:
* Tame fly away hair
* Manage frizzy hair
* Untangle your hair
* Leave curly hair smooth and silky

How often should you have a leave-in hair oil treatment

You apply leave in conditioner after shampoo or rinsing to manage those hard to tame curls so you can use it as often as needed.

<u>Recipe 1</u>

Detangler leave in conditioner

INGREDIENTS:
- 5 tablespoon of distilled water
- 1 tablespoon of aloe vera gel
- 10 drops of rosemary essential oil
- ½ to 1 tablespoon vegetable glycerin

PREPARATION:
1. Place the aloe vera gel on a glass spray bottle.
2. Pour in the distilled water.
3. Add the vegetable glycerin.
4. Add the rosemary essential oil drops (you can also use lavender).
5. Cover the bottle and shake to mix until the the aloe vera gel dissolves.

APPLICATION:
* Wet hair.
* Spray on the mix to help untangle your hair.
* Allow it to set in for a minute.
* Brush your hair to remove the tangles.

STORAGE:
Keep in a spritz sprayer

SHELF LIFE:
Because of the water content, bacteria could set in so it is best to make a one application recipe.

Recipe 2

. . . .
Creamy leave in conditioner
. . . .

INGREDIENTS:
- 1 oz softened coconut oil
- 2 oz aloe vera gel
- 1 teaspoon avocado oil

PREPARATION:
1. Combine all ingredients in a mixing bowl.
2. Using an electric mixer, mix all ingredients until consistency becomes thick and creamy.

APPLICATION:
* Wet hair.
* Apply the creamy mixture on your hair.
* Comb your hair until the mixture is evenly spread on your hair.

STORAGE:
Store in a cool dry place

SHELF LIFE:
Up to 2 applications.

Chapter 6
DIY Herbal Oil Infusion Recipe for Scalp Care Treatment

A healthy hair starts with a healthy scalp.

Your hair is like plants on a bed of soil, the soil being your scalp. Plants flourish on rich soil, if the soil is dry the plants get dry and eventually die.

In this chapter, you will find some DIY recipes to help treat your scalp and remove dandruff.

DRY SCALP TREATMENT

When your scalp is dry, it affects the growth and health of your hair so you need to treat your scalp as much as you treat your hair.

What is Dry Scalp treatment?

Dry scalp treatment is simply nourishing your scalp with the use of massage oil.

Severe cases of the dry scalp can cause skin inflammation often characterized by redness, itchiness, and flakiness.

Benefits of using dry scalp oil treatment:

Severe dry scalp can lead to a more serious problem than just dandruff and flakiness.

Often, chemical-based hair care products are the root cause of your dry scalp so it is best to use naturally based treatments such as oil. Here are some benefits of using oil treatment for dry scalp:

* Nourishes and hydrates your scalp.
* Helps balance the sebum in you scalp.
* Keeps your hair healthy and strong.
* Natural homemade oil treatment allows you to treat your scalp in the comfort and privacy of your own home.

How often should you have a dry scalp oil treatment

Treat your scalp to an oil massage at least 2 times a week.

Recipe 1

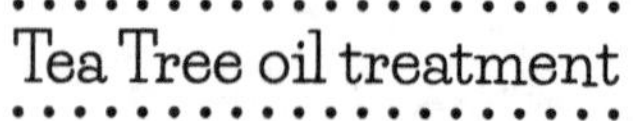

INGREDIENTS:
   • 1 oz Extra virgin olive oil
   • 1 – 2 drops of Tea Tree essential oil

PREPARATION:

1. Mix the olive oil and the tea tree oil in a jar.

2. Shake well.

APPLICATION:

* Apply the mixture onto your scalp directly.
* Massage your scalp while spreading the mixture.
* Gently comb your hair to remove some of the flakes.
* Leave it on for about 30 minutes.
* Rinse and shampoo your hair.
* Repeat the process after 2 days.

STORAGE:

Store in a dry cool place

SHELF LIFE:

Shelf life depends on the shortest shelf life of the oil you used

Recipe 2

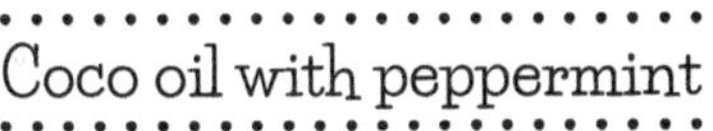

INGREDIENTS:

- 1 oz of coconut oil
- 2 drops of peppermint essential oil

PREPARATION:

1. Dilute the peppermint oil with coconut oil in a jar.

2. Shake well until they mix together.

Application:
  * Apply the mixture onto your scalp directly.
  * Massage your scalp while spreading the mixture.
  * Gently comb your hair to remove some of the flakes.
  * Leave it on for about 30 minutes.
  * Shampoo hair and then rinse thoroughly.
  * Repeat the process after 2 days.

Storage:
  Store in a dry cool place

Shelf life:
  Shelf life depends on the shortest shelf life of the oil you used.

Recipe 3:

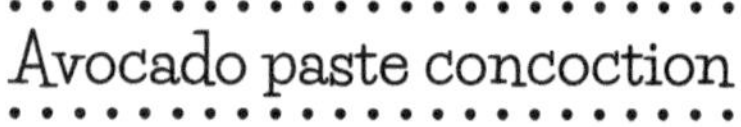

Ingredients:
  • Small ripe avocado
  • 2 tablespoon olive oil
  • 1 teaspoon honey

Preparation:
  1. In a mixing bowl, mash the ripe avocado until it becomes a paste.
  2. Add the olive oil and the honey.
  3. Mix well.

APPLICATION:
  * Apply the avocado paste on your scalp.
  * Gently massage your scalp.
  * Leave the mixture on your scalp for 30 minutes.
  * Rinse and shampoo your hair.

STORAGE:
  Do not store because the avocado will spoil.

SHELF LIFE:
  Good for one application only.

ITCHY SCALP TREATMENT

Itchy scalp is caused by dry scalp that can lead to dandruff.

White flakes on your black dress can be embarrassing. To avoid dandruff, you should treat it as early as possible.

Benefits of using itchy scalp treatment

Here are some the benefits of treating itchy scalp:

  * Removes itchiness and redness
  * Avoid early hair loss
  * Avoid embarrassing moments
  * Prevents dandruff

How often should you use an itchy scalp oil treatment

Use the treatment 2 times a week or as often as needed.

<u>Recipe 1:</u>

. . . .
Tea tree oil plus olive oil
. . . .

INGREDIENTS:
- 1 tablespoon olive oil
- 3 drops tea tree essential oil

PREPARATION:
1. Mix olive oil and tea tree oil together.

APPLICATION:
* Apply on your scalp spreading over your hair.
* Leave it on for 30 minutes.
* Comb your hair to remove the flakes.
* Rinse and shampoo your hair thoroughly.
* Repeat the process 2 to 3 times a week.

STORAGE:
Keep in dry cool place away from heat

SHELF LIFE:
Up to 2 applications.

<u>Recipe 2:</u>

Rosemary Oil infusion for itchy scalp and dandruff

INGREDIENTS:
- 1 cup virgin coconut oil
- 3-4 sprigs fresh rosemary leaves
- 6 drops rosemary essential oil
- 6 drops tea tree essential oil
- 6 drops lavender essential oil
- 5 drops patchouli essential oil
- ½ cup raw apple cider vinegar
- 1 cup water

PREPARATION:

For the infused oil:

1. Wash the fresh rosemary.

2. Place the rosemary on a towel and let it air dry. Make sure the herb is completely dry to avoid water moisture that can make your oil rancid.

3. In a double boiler, mix the rosemary leaves and the coconut oil.

4. Infuse for 2 hours on a slow heat.

5. Simmer and stir occasionally.

6. Pour the infused oil into a jar with a strainer on top.

7. Strain the rosemary leaves and discard.

8. Let it cool for 5 minutes.

9. Add all the essential oil and mix.

For the apple cider:

1. Dilute the apple cider with one cup of water.

APPLICATION:
  * Scoop the infused coconut oil with your fingers.
  * Apply the mixture to your roots and scalp.
  * Go over your entire head until your scalp and roots are completely soaked with mixture.
  * Massage your scalp as you go.
  * Apply whatever remaining infused oil to your hair ends.
  * Put up your hair in a bun and cover it with a shower cap or a towel.
  * Let it sit for 45-60 minutes.
  * Rinse your hair with clear water to remove the oil.
  * Shampoo and condition your hair after rinsing.
  * Pour the diluted apple cider on your scalp
  * Massage your scalp.
  * Rinse your hair thoroughly again.
  * Repeat the process 2 to 3 times a week.

STORAGE:
The recipe is designed for one application but if you made a lot, divide the mixture and store it in a cool dry place

SHELF LIFE:
Should last as long as the oil with the shortest shelf life.

Chapter 7
DIY Herbal Oil Infusion Recipe for Hair Problem Treatment

Hair problems are often caused by chemical based hair products, prolonged exposure to the sun and lack of proper hair care.

Whatever the reason, we have included in this chapter the most common hair problems that you encounter and listed homemade recipe treatments to deal with them.

DRY/HEAT DAMAGED HAIR TREATMENT

Dry hair is characterized by dull, frizzy, and lifeless stands. Dry hair happens due to the lack of moisture in your hair.

Dry hair often leads to hair damage like split ends and brittleness.

Shampoo residues can leave your hair dry and heavy. Daily styling and hair drying can also cause your hair to dry and get damaged. You can treat dry hair easily with a few simple DIY recipe.

What is dry hair treatment?

Dry hair treatment is giving back life and nourishment to your hair. Hair needs moisture to be healthy and strong.

If dry hair is not treated, it could lead to other hair damage problems like loss of hair.

Benefits of using dry hair oil treatment

Some of the benefits of treating dry hair are:

* Brings back vibrancy to your hair.
* Makes your hair strong and healthy.
* Makes your hair more manageable.

How often should you have a dry hair oil treatment

Your hair needs regular nourishment. A weekly conditioning will help a lot in restoring the natural oils on your hair.

Recipe 1:

Aloe Vera Gel Treatment for balanced pH level

INGREDIENTS:
- 1 Aloe Vera leaf
- ½ cup coconut oil
- 5 drops of rosemary essential oil

PREPARATION:

1. Cut the Aloe vera leaf.
2. Scrape off the fresh aloe vera gel and place it in a bowl.
3. Add the coconut oil.
4. Heat the mixture over low heat for 5-7 minutes.
5. Let it cool down completely.
6. Add the drops of rosemary.
7. Mix and then pour in a lid covered jar.

APPLICATION:

* Take the desired amount of oil for your hair.
* Slightly warm the oil.
* Apply the oil from the roots of your hair working towards the ends.
* Massage for 2 minutes in your scalp to stimulate blood circulation.
* Let it sit for an hour on your hair.
* Rinse and use a mild shampoo and conditioner.
* Repeat the process two times a week.

STORAGE:

Dark cool place

SHELF LIFE:

2 weeks

Recipe 2:

Onion Hair Oil (Sulfur-rich)

INGREDIENTS:
* 1 small sized red onion
* 2 cloves garlic
* 6 tablespoon coconut oil
* 3-4 drops lavender essential oil (you can also use rosemary)
* 1 teaspoon lemon juice
* Mug of water

PREPARATION:

For the oil mixture:

1. Combine finely chopped onion, garlic, and coconut oil in a small pan.
2. Heat the mixture in extremely low flame until it stops bubbling.
3. Let it cool down completely.
4. Add the drops of lavender essential oil.
5. Pour the oil in a glass bottle and strain.

For the lemon rinse

1. Mix lemon juice with the water to dilute.

APPLICATION:
* Massage the oil into your scalp lightly.
* Wrap your head with hot towel.
* Let the oil soak your hair for 20 minutes.
* Rinse, shampoo and condition your hair.
* To remove the smell of onion, use diluted lemon juice as final rinse.

STORAGE:
Sstore the oil mixture in a jar and refrigerate

SHELF LIFE:
10 days

Recipe 3:

Protective Oil for Heat Damaged Hair

INGREDIENTS:
* 1 tablespoon castor oil
* ¼ cup coconut oil
* 2 tablespoon avocado oil
* 10 drops rosemary essential oil

PREPARATION:
1. Combine all oil in an 8 oz covered jar.
2. Shake well to mix the oils.

APPLICATION:
* Scoop 1 tsp to 1 tbsp oil at a time.
* Rub the oil on your fingertips.
* Massage the oil into your scalp and hair starting from the roots to the ends.
* Let it sit overnight.
* Shampoo and then rinse thoroughly.

STORAGE:
Keep in a dry cool place

Will last the same time as the oil that has the shortest shelf life

GRAY HAIR TREATMENT

Premature graying can be a source of embarrassment to some.

You can delay gray hair by following some of this homemade organic recipe concoctions.

What is Gray Hair treatment?

Gray hair treatment is done either to delay gray hair or to cover gray hair.

Once your hair starts to gray, you can use organic herbs and oils to cover the graying.

Benefits of using Gray hair oil treatment

* Delay hair graying
* Bring back the natural color of your hair without the aid of chemical based hair colors
* Prevent hair loss

How often should you have a Gray hair oil treatment

Treatment should be 2 to 3 times a week

Recipe 1:

. . . .
Coco Curry Oil treatment
. . . .

INGREDIENTS:
- 1 cup coconut oil (about 8 oz)
- Bunch of curry leaves

PREPARATION:
1. Wash the curry leaves thoroughly.
2. Air dry the leaves to remove any moisture.
3. In a double boiler, boil water then reduce the heat to a simmer.
4. In a heat proof container combine coconut oil and curry leaves.
5. Infuse for a couple of hours, stirring occasionally.
6. Pour the oil in a glass covered jar and strain the leaves.
7. Let it cool for a few minutes.

APPLICATION:
* Apply the curry infused oil to your scalp.
* Massage your scalp gently.
* Let it sit for a few hours or overnight.
* Rinse and shampoo.

STORAGE:
Keep the mixture in a cool dry place

SHELF LIFE:

Coconut oil lasts more than 2 years and if your mixture has no moisture, it will not go rancid fast.

Recipe 2:

Fresh Aloe Vera Mask

INGREDIENTS:
  • Fresh Aloe Vera

PREPARATION:
1. Split open the Aloe Vera plant.
2. Scrape off the Aloe Vera gel.

APPLICATION:
  * Apply the fresh aloe vera gel directly onto your scalp.
  * Spread it from the roots of your hair to the tips.

STORAGE:

Keep the fresh aloe vera refrigerated.

SHELF LIFE:

Lasts more than six months to a year if refrigerated

Recipe 3:

. . . .
Sesame Oil with Henna
. . . .

INGREDIENTS:
- One cup of sesame oil
- Bunch of henna leaves

PREPARATION:
* Wash the henna leaves thoroughly.
* Air dry the leaves to remove any moisture.
* In a double boiler, boil water then reduce the heat to a simmer.
* In a heat proof container combine sesame oil and henna leaves.
* Infuse for a couple of hours, stirring occasionally.
* Pour the oil in a glass covered jar and strain the leaves.
* Let it cool for a few minutes.

APPLICATION:
* Apply the henna infused oil to your scalp.
* Massage your scalp gently.
* Let it sit for a few hours or overnight.
* Rinse and shampoo.
* Use it daily.

STORAGE:
Keep in a covered jar container storing in a dry cool place.

SHELF LIFE:
More than a year if without moisture.

HAIR LOSS TREATMENT

Hair fall naturally occurs to rid our hair of dead follicles but excessive hair loss is a problem.

What is Hair Loss treatment?

Hair loss treatment is simply using organic oil based treatments to restore hair growth and stimulate the hair follicle.

Benefits of using hair Loss oil treatment

Some of the benefits of hair loss oil treatment are:

* Stimulates blood circulation in the scalp
* Stimulates the hair follicle for hair growth
* Brings back the luster in your hair
* Prevent excessive shedding of hair

How often should you have a hair loss oil treatment
As often as necessary

Recipe 1:

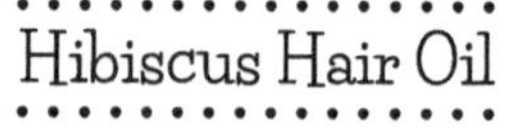

INGREDIENTS:
- 2 Hibiscus flowers
- ½ cup Hibiscus leaves
- ¼ cup coconut oil
- ¼ cup badam oil

PREPARATION:
1. Wash the hibiscus flower and leaves in cool water.
2. Sun-dry the hibiscus to remove all traces of moisture.
3. In a heatproof bowl, place the hibiscus flower and leaves.
4. Pour the coconut oil and badam oil.
5. In a double boiler, place the heat-proof bowl.
6. Keep the fire in low heat.
7. Infuse the oils and the hibiscus for 5 minutes.
8. Strain the oil after the infusion in a clean bottle.

APPLICATION:
* Take the desired amount of oil for your hair.
* Slightly warm the oil.
* Apply the oil from the roots of your hair working towards the ends.
* Massage scalp for about 2 minutes to stimulate blood circulation.
* Let it sit overnight for better absorption.
* Rinse and shampoo the next day.

STORAGE:
Store in a clean jar

SHELF LIFE:
Should last for more than a year as long as there is no moisture in the oil.

Recipe 2:

Ginger Ayurvedic Hair oil

INGREDIENTS:
- 1 tablespoon grated ginger
- ½ cup olive oil
- 3 drops rosemary essential oil

PREPARATION:
* Heat olive oil in extremely low heat.
* Add the grated ginger.
* Let the oil and ginger boil until the moisture evaporates.
* Let the oil cool.
* Filter the oil and pour in a dark glass bottle.
* Add the drops of rosemary essential oil.
* Shake to mix all the ingredients thoroughly.

APPLICATION:
* Apply the mixture on your scalp and hair starting from the roots to the tips.
* Use your fingers to gently massage the oil.
* Let it sit for 15 minutes.
* Rinse in lukewarm water followed by a mild shampoo.
* If you have sensitive scalp, some properties of the ginger could cause mild irritation but it should fade after some time.
* If irritation persists, shampoo your hair thoroughly to remove all traces of the oil in your hair.

STORAGE:
Dark bottle in a dark cool place

SHELF LIFE:
2 weeks

Chapter 8
Making your Recipe — Your DIY Recipe Guide

Now that you know more about herbs, carrier oils, and essential oils you can now start making your own recipe.

In this chapter, I will make it easy for you to prepare your own concoction by providing you with a step by step guide and reference charts that you can use.

I have classified each oil category based on the benefits that your hair will receive so that you can choose your oils easily.

YOUR HERBS AND ESSENTIAL OILS

This chart will include different kinds of herbs you can use either in its raw form or as an essential oil:

herbs	Body/ Luster	Hair Loss	Scalp	Gray- ing	Dry/ Dam- aged	Oily Hair	Dan- druff	Condi- tion	Anti Inflam- matory
Aloe Vera	X	X	X		X			X	
Amla		X	X		X			X	
Aritha	X	X	X				X		
Basil	X	X	X		X				X
Bhringraj		X		X	X		X		
Black Tea		X		X					
Burdoch			X		X	X	X	X	X
Calendu- la (Mari- gold)				X	X	X			
Chamo- mile			X	X		X			X
Curry				X					
Henna	X			X	X			X	
Lavender	X	X	X				X		X
Nettle	X	X	X		X	X	X		
Pepper- mint		X	X			X			X
Rose- mary	X	X	X		X	X			X
Yucca Root		X	X		X		X	X	

YOUR CARRIER OILS

This chart includes the most commonly used carrier oils to dilute or infuse essential oils:

Carrier Oil	Scalp	Dry / Damaged	Oily	Shiny	Nourish	Hair Loss	Gray	Conditions
Jojoba Oil		X			X			
Coconut Oil	X	X		X	X			X
Olive Oil	X			X				
Sweet Almond		X			X			
Apricot	X		X			X		
Avocado	X	X			X			X
Argan		X		X				X
Grape-seed	X		X	X	X			
Hazel Nut	X	X			X			
Sesame	X	X			X		X	

YOUR DIY PROCEDURE

A step by step guide on how to prepare your own infused oil.

Step 1 - Choosing your treatment

The first step is to choose what type of treatment you want to prepare. Do you want a deep conditioner, a pre poo, or treat damaged hair?

The best treatment to start with is a deep conditioner or pre-poo and a light conditioner you can use and carry.

Deep conditioner treatments give the most number of benefits to the hair. A deep conditioner can address both scalp and hair problems.

Step 2 - Choosing your herbs and essential oil

Choose the best herb that would address your requirement. There are plenty of herbs to choose from.

You can combine fresh herbs and drops of essential oil to your recipe, just make sure you will dilute both with a carrier oil.

In this example, you can choose Aloe Vera for your deep conditioning, mixed with burdoch essential oil.

For your light conditioner treatment, use Yucca root mixed with either lavender or rosemary. In this example let us choose lavender. Yucca root has cleansing properties that are good for the hair.

Step 3 - Choosing your carrier oil

Carrier oils help dilute essential oils extracted from herbs. The carrier oil softens the harsh properties of your herbs.

Coconut oil is best mixed with aloe vera as part of your deep conditioning mixture. Coconut oil also help treat your scalp and nourish your hair.

For your light conditioner, you can choose sesame oil as your carrier to dilute your essential oil.

Step 4 - Preparing your infusion

When preparing your infusion, make sure that you do it subject it to extremely low heat, otherwise it will destroy your oils.

Use of a double boiler is suggested so that your mixture will be steam heated instead of direct flame heated.

Step 5 - Storing your mixture

Always store your mixture in a sterilized lid covered jar and place it in a dry cool place away from sunlight.

Some mixtures require refrigeration for storage.

In this sample, you can use a bowl for your deep conditioner because application will be done using your fingers. It is easier to scoop the mixture if the mouth of your container is wide.

For your light conditioner, turn it into a leave in conditioner. You can place it in a spritzer so you can carry it around and spray on when needed.

Step 6 - Applying your mixture

Apply your oil treatment based on the extent of your hair damage. A more extensive damage would require application often, perhaps even daily.

For maintenance, it is safe to apply it once a week.

Your Recipe

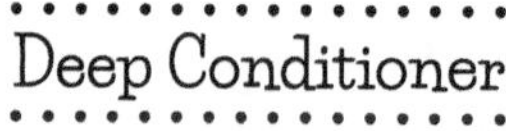

INGREDIENTS:
- 2 Aloe Vera
- 1 cup coconut oil
- 10 drops argan oil

PREPARATION:
1. Cut open the Aloe Vera.
2. Scrape off the aloe vera gel onto a heat proof mixing bowl.
3. Pour in the coconut oil.
4. Mix the aloe vera gel and coconut oil until the mixture turns into a thick consistency.
5. Add the argan oil.
6. Heat the mixture in a double boiler until it becomes warm.

APPLICATION:
* Scoop the thick mixture using your fingers.
* Massage the mixture into your scalp.
* Apply more mixture on your hair starting from the roots towards the ends.
* Let it set in for an hour or overnight for deeper absorption.
* Rinse and shampoo the next day.

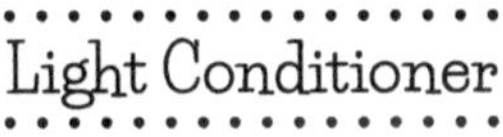

Light Conditioner

INGREDIENTS:
* 1 piece yucca root
* ½ cup sesame oil
* 1 tablespoon avocado oil
* 2-3 drops lavender essential oil

PREPARATION:
1. On a double boiler under extremely low heat, infuse the yucca root with ½ cup of sesame oil.
2. After 5-7 minutes, remove the infusion and let it cool completely.
3. Pour into a spritzer and strain the root.
4. Add the avocado oil.
5. Add the lavender essential oil.
6. Close the spritzer and shake the mixture well.

APPLICATION:
* Spray the mixture on your damp hair (after washing).
* Spread the mixture from roots to the tips.
* Comb your hair to remove the tangles.
* Leave the mixture on your hair until your next washing day.
* As needed, you can spray on the mixture on your.
* Rinse and shampoo on your next washing day.
* Repeat the process.

Conclusion

Hair care business is a huge industry, just looking at the statistics presented in this book. It continues to grow every year. This proves the importance we give to our hair.

The good news is that manufacturers are now investing heavily in the use of organic-based ingredients. This will give the growing number of consumers who are switching to organic products.

Sadly, the hair care segment industry is a money maker and manufacturers will try to recover the huge amount they invested on R&D. This will make the organic hair care products be more expensive.

This is why I wrote this ebook.

I want to address the problem of people who are looking for organic products which are not costly.

The information in this book aims to give people a chance to use organic products using a variety of ingredients that they can easily find in their kitchen or in the supermarket.

The ingredients listed here are mostly garden variety and will not be hard to find.

This book arms the average consumer with an arsenal that they can use to combat the issue of hair and scalp problems.

A healthy, shiny hair is not a just a dream. It can be a reality even for the average consumer.

For more tips, you can visit my website and social media accounts:

Website: https://www.clishea.co

Pinterest: https://www.pinterest.com/beclishea

Facebook: https://www.facebook.com/beclishea

Instagram: https://www.instagram.com/beclishea

THANK YOU AND GOOD LUCK!

www.ingramcontent.com/pod-product-compliance
Lightning Source LLC
Chambersburg PA
CBHW060756260726
48660CB00002B/653